Be The Best You Can Be.
(polio my constant companion)

ISBN-13: 978-1478122319
ISBN-10: 1478122315

Introduction:

This book covers one person's story of life with this virus, and the effects it had on his life. There are many I am sure, stories from people living with this, or from people who know someone who has survived polio. This account is written in the victim's own words, as he lived it and viewed his life. It is a personal account.

It is hoped that this book shows a lighter side to the personality of the sufferer as well as the obvious challenges that presented themselves throughout his life, and will continue to do so.

For those who have suffered the effects of polio, you will already be aware of the reality of the change it makes to life. For those who are just taking an interest in the subject you may be surprised to learn there are many ways this can affect the human body.

Depending on the virus type, the effects can range from nothing noticeable in around 95% of cases, to paralysis, where the virus enters the central nervous system and by infecting motor neurons, destroys them which in turn leads to muscle weakness and paralysis. The most common type of paralysis is from spinal polio, which more often affects the legs. There is no cure, there is only a vaccine to protect you.

For survivors, there is always the ticking time bomb (maybe an exaggeration) of PPS. This is 'post polio syndrome', and can affect survivors of polio around forty years after recovery from the original infection. Again, there is no cure for this, and although it is not generally life threatening, symptoms can include progressive weakness and muscle deterioration, joint pain and fatigue.

People in recent history of note, which most will at least know the name of, who suffered from this condition, include US President Franklin D. Roosevelt, reportedly contracting the virus whilst swimming in a lake in Canada and was left permanently paralysed from the waist down, and singer Ian Drury, who believed he contracted it from a swimming pool in Essex, England, when he was seven.

Preface :

If you are expecting a read that is full of anger, and blame and depression, then you will be disappointed. This book is an outline of the life of one survivor of this virus, and the legacy that remains after survival. It is hoped that it will encourage others with this, or other afflictions to see that there is always a life to be led. It may be far from the life you may have wished for, or indeed the life you might choose, but it is still a life.

This story has not reached a conclusion as yet, as there may well be hurdles to jump in the future, but for now this is the living history.

Be The Best You Can Be (polio my constant companion)

Be The Best You Can Be.
(polio my constant companion)
As narrated by Michael B.

Shall I write this or not? was the immediate question. I guess if you are reading this then the question answers itself. Just another person's story that has so much meaning to the person in question, but would there be an interest in another's personal history?

Having survived polio and heart disease, two heart attacks and a few accidents along the way, not totally unscathed, and being now nearer the end of the road than the beginning, maybe it is time to share the fact that life may have had its fair share of ups and downs, but on the whole has remained a rewarding experience.

Life started out in 1956 at Hunter Road on RAF Thorney Island. At that time in Emsworth Hampshire, mum was a nurse and dad of course was in the RAF serving as a corporal, following the normal practice in the UK then, of conscription into the forces. Santa Clause would arrive by helicopter which, from a child's perspective, had some excitement to it. Our family lived there for just a few years before moving to Littlehampton, a seaside town in Sussex. Dad would then commute to work, but was not seen for months on end due to overseas postings when my sisters and I were small.

Before our move from the base, we as a family, my parents and two sisters, spent some time in Yemen, based at RAF Khomaksar. Square concrete block buildings, white to reflect some of the heat and more sand outside than you could shake a stick at. The beaches were fenced off to keep everyone out of the sea, thus avoiding us becoming shark bait. We had a 'house boy' as he was referred to, and was employed to do simple tasks around our quarters. There was one occasion we arrived at our quarters to find the termites had been active, to the extent that the stair case had collapsed!

Entertainment was limited here, with the 'BBC world service' via the radio, camel racing being a regular highlight, this entertainment provided by Yemeni locals, and indeed the excitement of car racing around the buildings was not unknown.

It was here in Yemen that my life changed. I was always told that I had fallen from a second storey window, and never thought to pry further as the years went by. My resulting visit and stay in hospital there to fix a broken leg, dealt me a blow to live with and to overcome as life went along. An infection of polio at the hospital whilst being treated for the bone break, resulted in the paralysis of the same leg, and having started walking at one year old, had now to learn the art once again. I have no recollection of ever being able to walk unaided. There would be another occasion that I had to learn this basic in later years, but that is a long way off at this time.

Surviving the fall with a broken leg was lucky, but the broken leg was the weakness. Unable to walk on it, by the time it had healed the damage the virus had caused was irreversible. Personally, it was a very expensive fall, the cost of which would remain with me every day of my life from this point.

Life in general was pretty good, my father always worked hard to improve life for us. From the days of moving from the base, I remember probably the same as most others in the late 50's and early 60's, the days before wall to wall carpets and central heating, there were rugs on the floor and we had a paraffin heater in the bedroom I shared with my eldest sister, her on the top bunk, me below, and my younger sister sleeping in a cot in my parents room.

I do remember when we first returned from Yemen, where my younger sister on one occasion had sat on a termites nest and got badly bitten, there were problems getting her to wear any clothes at all as she had never worn any before having spent pretty much all of her first year in Yemen. Dad had an RAF motorcycle he used to get to work at the side of the house, though sometimes he would use an RAF Commer van, RAF blue with the usual RAF motif on each side. Looked very smart in its day! I remember one time travelling back to our house with dad and a colleague of his, me sitting on the heater of the commer van which was situated between the two front seats and became quite warm. I did fall asleep on the way back from Thorney Island where we had set out from, but it was nice to get time away from my sisters who were at home with mum, and have some time with the adults even though I was probably taken along to give mum some time to do girlie things with my sisters.

My mother used to say that at least I would not be asked to fight for my country, (usually when there was a news item on the radio or television regarding some military action overseas) maybe this is one of the things that assisted in my estrangement from her. We never really got on which is a little sad, but I felt strongly that I wanted the same options to choose what I wanted from life as any other child would have, and did find new frustrations to overcome as I grew in years. These feelings of wanting freedom of choice were there from very early years, and remained with me always.

There was one time I remember when I was around five years old, I was crying in my bed. My father came in to see me, sat beside me and asked what was wrong. He questioned whether I was being bullied at school. I had no answer for him apart from that was not the case. I dried my tears pretty quickly and told him I was fine. The fact was, I was hating my situation. I was young, I did not understand many things, but from time to time I would question why I was different. That 'why me?' moment. That was my only reason to be upset. If I had had an older head on my shoulders, I would have discussed it with him, but I think he knew how I felt.

These early years of walking were aided by a full leg splint with no means to bend the leg at the knee when sitting. This was uncomfortable but was something I had no control over as this was the only option available to me. I felt clumsy, restricted, and far from the same as everyone else.

Recalling what is remembered as many hours at hospital waiting rooms waiting to see a bone specialist, in those days was being in a long hallway, with over thirty other patients waiting for various reasons. Every time the nurse would come out to call a name, there was the hope that it was my name she would call. They were never anywhere near the time of the appointment allocated, and so you would sit, wait, get bored out of your brain staring at the plain walls and inhaling the clinical smell of the corridor. This was a regular occurrence, and as a child I never understood why so many visits, nor why it always took so long.

Nothing ever changed, and despite my asking questions and receiving vague promises from the surgeon, ie: "we may be able to do something when you get older" (which I recall actually did give me some hope for the future when I was eleven) the fact remained, nothing ever did change. These visits were always with my mother. She never asked him any questions. I guess she knew. She would refer to me as an 'awkward' child, she never knew how awkward I felt at times during that period of my life.

I think dad was sad to leave the RAF when his option to leave came, and there's a question I should have asked, but never did get the opportunity, why did he choose to leave? I probably know the answer and have to guess that pressure from home was the reason.

Mum was never really the touchy feely type of person towards any of the children. I am not sure where her perspective came from, and whilst her mother, my grandmother, was not 'overly' affectionate, she did always find time to get involved with us as kids. Whenever we spent time with her she would always be happy to get out the Monopoly board or a pack of cards, or even sit at her kitchen table and 'glue stuff' or make things with us. Taking the time to explain things, and never a cross word and always considerate towards us. I always appreciated her willingness to explain rather than dictate. I certainly learned a lot from her over the years, and perhaps her living in London during the blitz, had encouraged her in turn to encourage us to watch factual programmes about world war two on the television when we were at her house. I found this history very interesting and probably learned more from these programmes than I did from History lessons at school.

From this first small house we moved to a three bedroom semi about a mile away, that was to be home until I was twelve years old. It was like our first house on a nice quiet road, and dad went to work for the Hoover company. Now the girls had their own room to share, and mine was pretty nice with a work area dad built for me to make all the Airfix models that I enjoyed making. Mostly aircraft, surprisingly! Dad would often find some time to help also. He was always busy, but somehow always managed to find some time for me as well. He would never let me win at draughts which taught me that in a game the winner is the better player. From this I hope I managed to learn to do the best I could do, and be the best I can be, but often felt I had to 'outdo' others just to be noticed as otherwise I was seen as the odd one out and not worth the time of day. That is I guess how I felt a lot of the time as a youngster. I was to continue to learn as I travelled through life, that competition was always around me. I would often look back at these days and feel encouraged to try just that little bit harder.

When it came to Christmas and birthdays there were only ever two items I wanted, an Airfix model kit or some new item for the railway. I think dad also enjoyed the train set too, which was good as I ended up with so much railway stock and track I felt like the king of the Great Western Railway! He even made an electric red and green light signal for my trains and taught me how to re-wire an electric motor.

We had an old upright piano in the front room which saw me after several lesson playing 'London's Burning' for my grandmother to listen to during her visits. I was never really any good with the piano and soon opted to stop taking the lessons much to the relief of the neighbours I am certain. I knew I was never going to be a classical pianist that is for certain, not even a Russ Conway or Rick Wakeman for that matter. It did not help that I had to sit side on to the piano as I was unable to bend my leg at this time, due to the fixed splint which was part of every waking moment if I wanted to be mobile.

It was here I was given my first set of wheels for one birthday, a push scooter! blue and yellow, and was my entertainment for that summer, spending most of the day enjoying using it. It had a brake pedal towards the rear of the footplate, and I managed to use it so much, I ended up with blisters on my feet. I never told anyone about this, but discovered if I soaked some toilet tissue in surgical spirit and put these soggy pieces of paper between my socks and my skin, they soon healed. I was more concerned my mother would say I could not use the scooter because of the damage I had caused myself, but this was my 'escape' and there was no way on earth I was going to allow any restriction to this little bit of freedom I had found.

There was one time when I was around ten, my parents arranged a magician to entertain for my birthday, and my friends from the neighbourhood were of course invited. Two of these friends lived across the road from us, two brothers, the eldest was a good pal and we used to play out in the summer, his younger brother however was the young pest, but he was invited also which is the right thing to do (as I remember being told). He however, spent most of the time saying 'it's up your sleeve' to the magician, which seemed to annoy the adults more than us kids all sat around in wonderment at this amazing man doing these tricks in our front room. I think the adults were hoping that the magician would wave his wand and make little Danny disappear! The best bit for me was when the magician made a cake appear as if from nowhere. That was one birthday to remember, and I always did.

There were many happy times at this house. I do remember scraping the ice off the inside of the window in my room there to look outside in the winter and seeing the telegraph lines sitting low under the weight of frost and snow. We never seemed to notice the cold in those days. The house had two fire places downstairs one in each of two rooms but only that in the living room would normally be lit. I think getting used to central heating in later years makes you notice the cold more, that and being less active of course. This however was the sixties and some luxuries in those days, had not become widely available as yet, such as central heating, double glazing and fitted carpets.

I spoke about my grandmother earlier, she was a typical 'old lady' grandmother, as kids we would often spend time at her house, either being baby sat or visiting as a family for lunch. She had a small-holding as a back garden, with chickens and ducks. On the right hand side of a pathway was a large caged area for the chickens and ducks. On the left were Bramley apple trees leading to three bee hives and a long metal shed along the bottom where she bred and kept rabbits for eating. I recall between the trees were stinging nettles, docks and purple foxgloves.

On one occasion I was out there walking around on my own and got to the rabbit shed and found a rat. Here was I, never having seen one before at around 4 or 5 years old, to me the closest thing I had seen to it was a hamster in a pet shop window. It felt really soft to stroke and it just stayed there, not attempting to run away or bite, just sat and let me stroke it!

Well, following my return to gran's kitchen and advising my mother that I had found a hamster in the garden. Panic!

Not from me of course. Looking back I think she thought I may have caught the plague, certainly used a lot of soap washing my hands that day!

Most of the time at her house was spent in the kitchen, especially in the winter, when she would have the fireplace burning and we would sit and watch as the flames made patterns on the back plate of the fire where the soot was. Here also she would fill our time making scrap books from, well, scrap really. Cutting up pictures from magazines and pasting them into books we made from card with her 'home made' glue. (water and flour). Simple things that kept us occupied. Then of course there was the Monopoly game which was probably my favourite pastime there.

Grandad used to just smoke a lot really, and whilst I think he was pleased to see us, he generally kept quietly to himself doing odd little tasks around the house. He did read a story to me on one occasion I remember having pestered him too! He also surprised me once, by taking me for a spin in his car, and driving close to the curb purposely to splash large puddles up into the air, which was quite entertaining. I think he quietly had a pretty good sense of fun.

We had just come back from a family holiday, when dad was told that he was being made redundant. What a blow for him. As kids we did not really feel the consequence at the time, but for him it must have been devastating. I do recall him saying if he had known before hand he would not have spent the money on that holiday. He always tried to do nice things for us as a family, we would often go to a theatre to see a play, probably something my parents wanted to see rather than for us kids, but from Camelot to the Black & White Minstrels Show in London, (which we had also seen on the television) they were all fascinating to me. We saw a few films too that nowadays would be taken for granted, but would not normally be on television for another twenty years, like Chitty Chitty Bang Bang, Help, The Sound of Music, in those days these were awesome days out.

Fortunately for us all, he soon had a new job that would see him and us through. He was employed by a family owned electrical company in Worthing, West Sussex, which already had a good local reputation and he was very successful there.

This gave the family the chance to move to a new house. This new house was amazing to me, we got to look around the house while the builders were still building it. Boy! was I in my element, and I could see the sea from my bedroom window. We moved during the school summer holidays after my final year at what was then called junior school, so me being twelve years old. Here myself and my sisters made many friends, and often, as we lived in a close the other kids would come to play outside with their bikes, scooters, space hoppers and pogo sticks etc.

It was at this time also that the hospital presented me with my first leg splint with a knee joint. It allowed me to unclip it when sitting which allowed a little more comfort and practicality.

I had never ridden a bike up to this point, only the scooter that I had a few years ago. I decided to experiment now at least I could bend my knee, and fortunately I managed to balance and pedal and stay upright first time. Actually this was exciting, I did not want to stop, I was pedalling, the bike was getting faster, and I was having a blast! Such a shame I had to give the bike back, but I knew I wanted a bike from that moment.

A deal had to be done. OK, so I get a paper round, so I can pay for new tyres, and repairs and handlebar mirrors etc. My grandmother got me a Raleigh bike. Metallic blue which looked even better after my first weeks paper round money having purchased some red and white tape to add to it. The added bonus of this transport was that I could now cycle the two miles to school, which was handy as it was the summer holidays when we moved and there was now quite a walk to the bus stop from this new house. These holidays were the best I can remember. So many days out on that bike, passing the time away cycling around what was now my new home town, discovering what shops we had and what they sold. Suddenly even friends that were a couple of miles away were just around the corner, as I could ride out to see them or meet them in the park, whereas I would never have walked all that way. Neither would they..but I was always grateful to gran for this bike.

As always, however long the summer seemed, it had to end and so back to school.

At senior school, we had to take a proficiency test in order to be allowed to cycle to school. On taking mine, one of those testing us came over to me and said "we are not supposed to teach people like you". Insulted? surprised? speechless? angry? just a little.

I thought it was only kids that were ignorant. I ignored him, pretending he had not made that statement, and continued doing as I was asked, and gained my certificate along with everyone else taking the test that day. Well it was hardly rocket science. You stay on, or you fall off, there was no in-between. Today I would be happy to confront him just to tell him what an ignorant twit he was that day. He did nothing for me that day, but to remind me of the differences between myself and the majority, and I was thirteen at this time and was just beginning to see how people can be. At the time it was another of those 'why me?' days.

The trip to school varied in levels of difficulty. Although most days were fine, the days when I had to pedal against a head wind were not so much fun. I was only able to push down on the pedal with one leg of course, as the other had no useable muscle, therein lay the issue, keeping the cycle in motion long enough for the pedals to go around one more time to repeat the process of pushing the pedal on one side down again. Sometimes this journey could take a little longer than other times, but it was always managed. When other kids might cycle past me on their way home, I would think quietly to myself 'bastard!' and then laugh, it was only a very slight anger at my situation, but it kept the adrenaline going to get me either to home or school and was forgotten once I had achieved my goal of arriving at whichever destination.

Senior school resulted in five years of exploring new things, from physics which I enjoyed the most to mathematics, which I struggled a little with until my final year when my teacher Mr Hampton was able to teach in a way that was not only interesting, but was made compelling and easy to understand. Thanks to him alone I managed that GCE. We had a woodwork teacher who had long hair and a moustache and carried around an acoustic guitar most of the time. He got the nickname Dylan, not after the popular singer, but was named after the rabbit on Magic Roundabout, a child's programme. He probably knew this but he never mentioned it. I do remember one exam we sat where we were supposed to write down the names of insects that do damage to wood, ie; death watch beetle etc, I added termites to my list which was marked wrong ? From this result he went down in my estimation despite that fact that he was a musician! These days I would have been able to tell him to 'google' it !

In those days I was able to leave school at fifteen, but stayed on an extra year to take the GSE exams, which were taken in the fifth form. In this year I received a small reward for writing, and was awarded to me for song lyrics that I used to write, and was encouraged and nominated by my then English teacher. The reward was in the form of a gift voucher for a local book store. These lyrics were for a couple of friends who had a band, but I enjoyed the writing, and so armed with a few basic chords put a few songs together for them. Prior to this with an old school friend James, I put together a pop magazine for school, more a case of a couple of sheets of A4 typed out for each copy as we had no access to any alternative devices, and it included a list of the current weeks charts. I remember clearly the first week was T.Rex with the song Hot Love at number one, which remained the case for several weeks. We sold these for around 3d each, (pre decimalisation) which would be around 1p in today's money, but surprisingly kids wanted to buy them.

The money of course went to pay for the next typewriter ribbon and paper.

On leaving school I made friends with a couple of lads, and was re-acquainted with another old friend from my younger years, Peter, and together we formed a band. It was of course the best rock band in town, being as the town was very small ! Peter was the true musician here, and could play almost any instrument given the time to practice it. His piano and guitar playing were fantastic. We only managed to play local gigs, and gained the use of the local church hall by way of ensuring we went to the church service on a Sunday evening. (before we went to the pub to play darts and bar billiards).

We always did however, manage to get a fair few to attend our gigs, and with homemade speaker stacks attached to our amplifiers, managed to put together quite good evenings without electrocuting ourselves. Me? the singer of the songs I wrote for us.

My mother would comment that she only ever knew what I was doing when she read the newspaper.

Never a shortage of girls in those days, one in particular managed to bring me out of my shell more than most, but she did draw attention arriving at one of the church services in a low cut short yellow dress with no bra. I think everyone in the congregation was talking about her that evening, her figure was shall I say well blessed....

I did have a pleasant but brief time chasing Martin's sister Sarah, but although she was intelligent company, and did kiss really well, I decided that this was not to be pursued long term, as I had always got on really well with the family and did not want to spoil my relationship with them all. The feelings at this time of confusion within myself, as to what 'others' would find acceptable were no doubt based on prejudices I had thus far encountered in my life, and so I was in a way trying to conform to what others expected of me. This decision at the time however, also enabled me to feel that I had not 'failed' on this occasion, as I had not tested how far this relationship could in reality go, and after all, I had made this decision. On reflection, and without my 'constant companion' I would have liked to have found out. This was a period in my life where the 'why me' was often very much present in my thoughts, and so it was actually affecting the decisions I was making.

Soon after this I met a girl called Melissa through the church, visiting from the United States with her parents. I introduced her to T.Rex music and in turn she introduced me to 'The Doors'. One haunting track which I love is entitled 'People Are Strange'. Mildly amusing music track, and words that I could associate with on a personal level. I actually thought a lot of her and we kept in contact by mail for some months following her return, but lost contact (for some years) soon after she returned home to Shawnee Mission, Kansas, due to circumstances in my private life, namely the death of my father.

It was two weeks before Christmas when we lost him. He was off work sick at the time, and in bed calling for help. I recall thinking right away this is not him. He never needed help. He was always there when he was needed. He was the 'helper' to us all. He was never sick let alone in need of assistance.

On entering the room, he told me he could not see. I called the doctor right away, and then called the store where my mother was working and told her she needed to come home.

The doctor duly arrived, as did my mother. The doctor stated that he did not consider that there was anything serious the matter, but did say that if we wanted to call an ambulance that would be ok.

My mother looked at me. She had never sought any advice from me, in fact she was the law maker at home. This one time, never to be repeated question in her eyes was startling to me, but easy to respond to.

This was the woman who had washed my mouth with soap because I had used the word damn at the age of nine. I had only ever heard my father use this word, probably when he hit his thumb with a hammer whilst doing a spot of DIY at home, and it did not seem that bad to me. I later learned that it was a common form of religious profanity, but as usual with my mother explanations were not something that took place, there was only HER way, no questions asked, literally..

I knew what she was asking me without her having to use any words. The woman I had a sense of fear of, was asking for my advice. No hesitation from me, "yes call the ambulance mum."

He was taken to a local hospital in Worthing, and was transferred to a London hospital within hours.

I was taken to visit him there on one occasion, to see him laying in a hospital bed with tubes everywhere, and he smiled as if to say he was pleased to see me. It was gratifying to know that he could see again, and although sad to leave the hospital, I had a sense that he was at least where he would be looked after, and 'repaired' and soon home as the father I knew.

That was the last time I was to see him. These were the darkest of days for me, but my tears were only ever seen by me.

Against all advice from doctors and relations, my mother refused an autopsy to take place, which of course left us all without any clue as to what he died of at the age of 42.

Mother only said at any time that she blamed his presence at the nuclear testing at Christmas Island for it, but a proven factual reason eluded all of those it affected. Christmas that year quite rightly never took place, and to some extent never felt the same again.

The band kept me focused on something I enjoyed, I needed it and it filled a space at the time. The friends I had within it helped me though this period of time.

There was also work to fill my days.

Taking the bus to work every day had become a tiresome chore, especially through the winter, but my grandmother came to the rescue and put down a deposit on my first bike as a birthday gift to me. It cost around £120, and I think the deposit was around £15. This was almost two weeks wages at the time, and I was already paying my mother £5 a week housekeeping, (around half my weekly wage in the early 1970's) so it made a major difference to me to just pay the insurance and the repayments each month. It gave me so much freedom also, as walking was limited for me, I could now visit my friends more easily, and more often.

I did manage to get pulled over for speeding a couple of times, and having resigned myself to the fact that a ticket and a fine would be issued, felt no shame in winking at a pretty girl on one occasion who was passing by as the police issued the ticket. It did seem to make the 'reward' for my haste a little less painful when she smiled.

A couple of the lads in the band had bikes too, Peter however made a point of winding up the local police on his!
He would ride up the High Street no hands, but worse than that, he would have not just his arms outstretched but his legs also, he was duly rewarded over a period of a few weeks with thirteen endorsements, which he became very proud of. It was quite easily achieved living as he did less than one hundred yards from the Police station.

Many days were spent with him at the home of his parents playing Beatles tracks, a little Credence Clearwater Revival and the Kinks, and adding some backing to these via the piano or guitar and working on songs.

Peter was the only one of us who made a career out of being a musician, and played mainly in Europe with his band at the time in later years. Sadly at the age of 27, he was to have a fatal heart attack whilst at home in Sussex with his family. He was talented, gifted, zany, great fun, intelligent admired and missed.

I had never really got on with my mother, we never did see eye to eye. I do have regrets about this, but try as I may, I felt that maybe in some way I was taking the blame for dad leaving the RAF. This will be an enduring question mark.
Things came to a head within a year of his death, and what with the cost of living at home and the restrictions on going out after work with my friends, I decided to try to make it on my own.

I put down a deposit on a bedsit, and made that home for now. I knew I could afford to do this from my wages, but did however forget that the cost of food and of putting coins in the electric meter, restricted my financial ability to go out with my friends of an evening. But at least I now felt the freedom I wanted had arrived, and I pretty soon learned to cook and was able to visit friends without permission or a time limit as to what time to be home. Looking back this was a good move for me. It felt like the right thing at the time and at one point I managed a full time and a temporary part time job to enable me to get the things I needed. I never did return home to live, and relied on myself from this relatively early age of sixteen. I may have lost the advantage of a cooked meal or washing done for me, but once again, I had found a 'freedom' or independence, which I was reluctant to give up.

I did later manage to get to college, studying accounting and book keeping. At last I was in an environment that I felt comfortable in. Like minded students, of similar ages, from many areas of the world. Not one person looked down on me, not one person appeared to see me as different. It was a great source of freedom to enjoy life also, and there were far more girls attending than lads. I took this opportunity to enjoy good female company in my free time, mainly watching movies at the cinema and, with John Travolta being king and Grease being 'the word' at this time, I had to see this movie several times. Each time of course having to say how enjoyable it was to see it! Fortunately, it was an enjoyable movie the first few times..

During my late teens, I became friends with a fellow who drove at weekends at a local grass track motor racing club in Angmering. From the first visit to watch this I was hooked on the noise, the dust, the smell of fuel and the adrenaline. I had to have a go. Managing to secure the purchase of an old car already set up for racing with the double harness and roll bars, my friend already advising that he was happy to take my car to the track each week, I was full of excitement. A couple of cans of household gloss paint changed it from blue to the 'Starsky and Hutch' livery seen below.

The car (with a manual gearbox) had gears and three pedals! ('Stick shift' for those reading this in some countries) ie, it was not automatic, which would prove a challenge with only the one leg suitable to push pedals down effectively.

With a little practice, I mastered how to make the thing go forward, twisting my foot around to cover more than one pedal at a time and missing a gear out here and there to save me having to change gear so often, although slowing down took a while to action, having to ensure I had found neutral before hitting the brake. The spring on the accelerator was changed for a weaker one which enabled me to use my restricted leg as a lever to push this down without too much effort. I did manage to get my racing licence having been able to convince the organisers that I was safe to race.

Getting in the car was also a challenge, as the doors were welded shut, and so the only route into the vehicle was through the passenger side window, the driver side having a protective grill across it as did the window at the front. All glass of course having been removed. I must have been quite pliable back then, and managed to get in more with the strength of my arms than anything else.

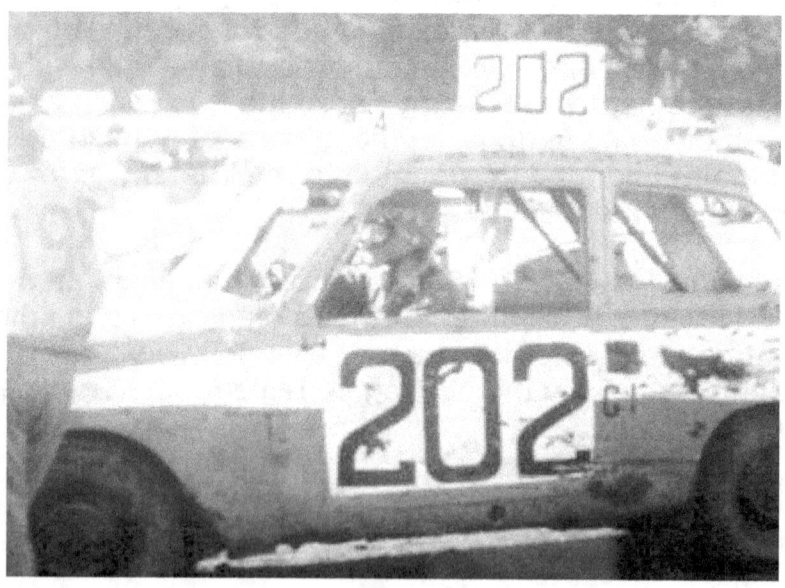

I would love to report here how well I did and how many races I won, but I did enjoy the racing. I found it very exciting, fast moving and it really did get the heart pumping. I managed to keep up pretty well, despite my lackluster gear changes, but in the end after a few weeks I managed to blow the engine. Well, that was a first anyway! This had been a real blast.

Teen years saw my passion for motorcycles continue until I was around twenty when I had decided that winter was not fun anymore and made the change to four wheels. This would prove to be a good thing as I was soon to find my dream job, working for an American Bank in the UK.

Apart from the challenges and good financial rewards, those being well earned I hasten to add, and not commission or bonus related, it allowed the financial freedom to travel that had not been available until this time. We had so many resources available at our fingertips. We had our own travel agency in the building for staff, our own bank, store and restaurant. I do not refer to a greasy spoon canteen, but the full scale real thing.

I had managed to trace a contact number for Melissa's father in Shawnee Mission, and was able to have a good chat with him, and having some time off coming up soon, decided it would be nice to make the trip over there.

Easy job, give our travel agent the dates I have and they did the rest. Flights booked and a return which allows me to travel from the airport to the office with time to spare to start work after my vacation. Sorted.

It all worked well. I spent some time in Ft Lauderdale following an invitation from my counterpart in our office in Florida. This was a great way to start the holiday.

My arrival at Miami International airport was not greeted, fortunately, with me going through a metal detector and being confronted by a group of alarmed and armed airport security officers, as the detectors were used on outward flights. I had realized naturally that they would be used to false alarms anyway, and so was prepared for a similar situation at some point. A quick check at arrivals was done with a hand held scanner to ensure most of me was in fact flesh and bone and not metal! However, it was the fact that I had arrived with only hand luggage, wearing a suit and tie, and also with a view to staying just a few days that led me to have to answer a few questions about my trip. The strangest thing was that having provided sight of my American Express card, the security officer advised "well if you have that with you, you will have no problems here," and having explained they were being vigilant due to the drugs trade, and reassuringly had accepted that I was neither a drug dealer nor a hit man, promptly wished me a good trip and apologised for any inconvenience.

January, hot, sunny, and I was treated so well and looked after so well, with sightseeing trips through to the Florida Keys amongst many trips out and about. It was with a little sadness I was to leave here as I was so well looked after by my host, for whom in just those few days I had grown quite fond of, and remain to this day eternally grateful to, but the next flight was to take me to Kansas City, which until now had been just a dream which I had held onto for many years.

Kansas, cold, minus 20ish! snow on the ground but I was amazed to see how they managed to cope over there. The snow routes were clear with the snow piled up alongside the roads. Seeing Melville again was brilliant. I had met him all those years ago, now thirteen years on I got to sit and chat with him once again.

We went to visit his daughter, my old friend Melissa and she invited me to stay with her family for my last few days. Her eldest daughter told me that her mother (Melissa) had informed her that I was very special to her mum. I felt very honoured to learn of this and admit I was very touched by her statement. She still had a copy of a vinyl album by T.Rex called 'Slider' which she had purchased way back when, following that introduction to it from me all those years ago. Melissa was married to a really nice guy and had three young daughters now. How things change when you are busy with life. I soon found out how to put weight on, with visits to various fast food chains! We had a great time catching up with all those years that had passed, and pretty soon it was time to return once more to the UK.

Melissa kindly arranged for her husband to take me to the airport for my return trip to London Heathrow. Whilst waiting for my return flight I decided to purchase a burger from a burger bar at Kansas City airport. I wanted to taste one more time that American beef which had enjoyed whilst over there. As I took my first mouthful, a cockroach meandered across the counter, and in an instant my appetite disappeared. I settled for a few glasses of whisky on the plane, followed by a long sleep.

One occasion I was in Kansas during my birthday and was given this rather scruffy and wonderful gift named Buzzy!

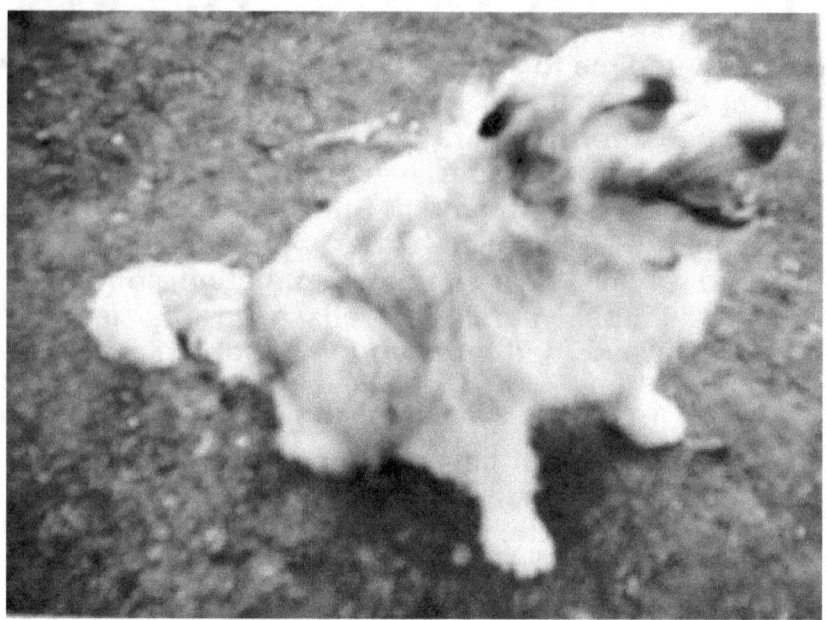

This was my birthday gift from Melissa and her family, and fortunately for me she and her family had planned to keep and take care of it, and so I had the pleasure of enjoying time with this dog when I was visiting without the time consuming effort of every day dog ownership. Best gift ever!

Life both 'over there' and over here was to me, perfect at this time, I expected this would continue.

Following several trips overseas thanks to my new found perfect jobs financial rewards, including a few trips back to Kansas, which for a few years became my 'second home', I was feeling a lot more adventurous and decided to add a new motorcycle to my options of transport. It was within just a few days of using this, I was to be involved in a collision which would change my direction in life.

On route to work one morning in June, one car driver decided to cut across my path leaving me no time to brake or avoid impacting my bike into her passenger side door. She later stated that she did not see me!! How often since have I heard people use that excuse. The result of the sudden impact sent me flying over the car. I remember everything happening so fast. I could only see in black and white and what I saw of the buildings passing past my view, were like freeze frame pictures with gaps rather than a fluid picture of what I could see. This was explained to me at the hospital later. I was advised that because things were happening suddenly and at a fast rate, my brain was unable to process all the information and so it was just processing what it could, hence the gaps and the lack of colour, apparently this was quite a common occurrence.

I landed on the road on the opposite side of the car to where my bike lay in ruins.

The pain was tremendous, until I sat up, and then it was gone. Regrettably this was not the end of the pain, or the problem, as I was to find out once the ambulance arrived.

The policewoman told me not to worry, the bike is fine. I am not sure what reply I gave to that, but at this moment I had no care about the bike, which was in fact written off. I guess she was trying to stop me worrying. I just asked her to call my office and to let them know I would be late and had an eagerness to be back at my desk!

I was told to lie down so they could pick up the stretcher, now this was the problem. The pain in my thigh would not allow me to lay down. I have to admit the ambulance crew, and the lady police officer at the scene, were so patient with me. It was following the x-ray that the problem was revealed. My bloody leg, being weakened from the polio all those years ago, shattered at the femur. Hence the pain as I tried to lie down and the parts of bone touched each other.

Following five days of being kept unconscious, and fifteen days after arriving at the hospital, surgery resulted in a metal plate being put in place to hold what parts they could use together.

Prior to surgery the kind policewoman who had stayed with me on the road at the site of the accident came to see how I was.
One thing she advised me took me straight back to the day I was taking my cycle proficiency test at school. Something I had not thought about in all these years. The driver of the offending vehicle had apparently tried to ease her own conscience having had time to think about it for a few days, and had told the police that she did not think 'people like me' should be allowed on the road. Deja-vu time for me...

I was assured however, that the police had told her in no uncertain terms how wrong she was. At the time with my leg in traction to keep the bones apart, I was feeling pretty helpless, but for just that moment I would have loved to have had the opportunity to face this idiot.

I was a lot tougher now than I was all those years ago. I had learned that some people do see an injury or unusual difference to a leg or an arm or a person in a wheelchair as somehow inferior and in some cases as lacking in ability to communicate or lacking in the ability to think for themselves. I have had many occasions to think, what if it's YOUR TURN next... as the result of perhaps a stroke, of a road accident or some other unavoidable occurrence?

These people, without a change in attitude, would never cope.

Here at the hospital, I mastered the art of wheelchair manoeuvring, and became quite expert at getting myself out and around the hospital without assistance, even managing a trip to a local store to buy cigarettes and spending a lot of time in the day room, which fortunately was also a smoking area. Then came the use of crutches, and a wheelchair would be no use in my two storey Victorian house. My arms were certainly getting stronger that was for sure, but I now had to learn to do things without having my hands free for a while, as the recovery I was informed was set to be some time off.

Back home took some adjusting. The hospital was an easy option, meals done and delivered, always someone there just in case, never needed but like an insurance policy, a reassurance, you knew the backup was there. Before the accident I would choose to either eat at the banks restaurant, or enjoy meals out with work colleagues. Suddenly things had changed and everything seemed alien to me.

Carrying a cup of coffee from the kitchen to the lounge using crutches? put cup on floor, sit down and scoot your backside along to the sofa moving the cup a little at a time until you reach your destination. The certainly was a learning experience.

I managed a few silly little jobs whilst recovering, even managed to wallpaper my downstairs hallway using a small set of steps, by getting myself up the steps on crutches whilst holding a length of paper at the same time. Managed to complete this without breaking my neck and was really pleased with the results. Health and safety? Hmmm .. it did however, take me a few days to do.

Some months on I felt good enough to return to work, but having spent so much time 'restrained' decided I wanted to have a holiday. I contacted my company who agreed this, and so I booked a week in Toronto Canada.

Annoyingly I did manage to break a couple of ribs from using the crutches a few days before my trip, but decided I would go anyway. This was a hard journey, but it was a sunny and very warm September in Toronto, and I was lucky to have work colleagues there to spend time with and trek out with. I managed to do the whole length of the annual exhibition there, a few miles long, on crutches, gave myself huge blisters in the palms of my hands, but they did not hurt, and by the time this vacation was over, my ribs were fixed and I felt great having had this escape for these few days. The leg was still tender and it was still a case of continue with the crutches, but with a little care not to knock it, it was not so bad.

I returned to work, only or a short while. I found it hard to concentrate at the time and eventually left in favour of starting my own business. It was sad to finish there, having spent so many years enjoying the job and the people I had worked with, not just locally but around the world.

I had an Italian girlfriend at the time of the accident, but she could not drive and I was not so adventurous to be out and about much at this point, so that came to an end. Her claim to fame was that of being an ex-fashion model, very small, pretty...and a great boost to my self esteem! To be fair, maybe it was my own vanity that encouraged me to enjoy her company.

Things were good when we could travel to see a show in the West End or spend evenings in a nice restaurant, but having stripped away the things we had both enjoyed at the time, there seemed little connection there. At least it ended on good terms.

Business grew by word of mouth, and was primarily transferring passengers to airports and docks. I actually ended up with my ex employer, the bank, putting me at the top of their list to call whenever they required a car to collect a visitor from or to go to the airport, not through anyone I knew, but from my solution to the first phone call they made to my company, they became a good customer. They were having difficulty getting transport to the airport at short notice, and wondered if I could help them. Well as it happened, all of my drivers were also busy on a motorway somewhere, and there was no option to re-route anyone to take the job. My solution was to offer them a free courtesy car, with no charge, and so I drove the passenger myself as a good will gesture as my company accepted their bank card as one form of payment that we took. Apparently, the lady passenger in question was quite high up the ladder and hence another company joined our growing list of professional customers. We managed to gain new custom on a regular basis from hotels, businesses, television companies, for example transferring actors across the country for film shoots. I put my heart and soul into this and managed to find time for only around 5 hours sleep a day, as I was determined to be available at the end of the phone at any time one of my cars was on the road.

The new venture was run from my lounge at home, which afforded me not only the luxury of watching movies in between incoming phone calls and dealing with the drivers of my vehicles, but saved a fortune in bills for business premises which were totally unnecessary and would have only been required, as I saw it, as an act of vanity, to have a 'high street' presence. This period of time is important to me as it was the first time I had felt totally free on constraints. Everything I did during this time was because I wanted to, because I enjoyed it, and there was nobody to tell me either 'it cannot be done' or 'you cannot do it like that'. I was totally committed to what I was doing, and it became almost an obsession. The job I had initially started up for 'me' had become an income which I was more than happy with.

The biggest advantage for me personally was that if I wanted to go out and drive I could, and if I was happier to stay at the end of the phone I had that option. It was good to be in control for this period of time.

Each vehicle would do 1,000 miles a week, and so there was the added continual booking in of servicing for the vehicles, to ensure they all kept running smoothly and also avoided being off the road being serviced when needed to take a passenger. Insurance and other documentation which all had to be kept up to date, and taking the bookings and payments were like another job to add to this, ensuring that not only did everyone get to where they needed to be on time, but were also collected on time. I also had the advantage of checking my cars every day when the drivers called in for their work lists for the following day.

We became so busy, that I made a decision to increase the charges to the customers, thinking this would cut down the amount of work coming in a little.

This decision was a failure, as far from decreasing, business just kept on rising. So, after five years of little sleep and total commitment, I decided to sell the business. This had been my own personal 'be the best you can be' but what started as a new dream job with total control, had become to some degree out of control, it was running away like an express train, a victim of its own success, and I was really feeling too weary to continue. It was a 'people' business, I knew my customers and they knew me. This was probably the nicest thing about it, but my energy had faded.

On reflection, this period of time would fit in with my personal 'PPS' due date (see introduction), but is not something I choose to concern myself with any more now than I did back then.

There was and still is the usual situation that the affected limb feels cold even in the summer, and the restrictions of the simplest thing like putting shoes on in the winter can take half an hour as your toes decide they want to bend downwards and refuse point blank to be dressed! and the tiredness of the hands, with a feeling almost of arthritis to the joints at times, which is just something annoying to work through until the pain goes.

Now it was time for some time out for a couple of months, which was spent sightseeing and travelling around the UK.

A few months after selling the business I realised maybe why that energy was no longer there. It may well have been the warning sign of what was to come next.

I awoke one night with extreme pain in the chest. My initial thought was that I had bad indigestion, but as the hours passed by and I felt worse, I became certain that I must instead have food poisoning somehow.

I began to feel freezing cold, at the same time however, sweet was pouring from my head, quite literally as it would from a tap, and I was feeling so tired I was increasingly anxious for this to end. A call was made for an ambulance, and I was advised, as they took me out of the house, that I was suffering a suspected heart attack.

Well that was not the worst thing I could have been told that night. 4 a.m. at the hospital in accident and emergency, a very caring lady doctor informed me that she had to give me a clot buster to break up the clot in the arteries around my heart. That sounded fine until she also informed me that whilst if she took no action then I would die without question, the effect of the clot buster may also lead to my death. Without it however I would not survive this night. I was then told that the decision was mine to make, as they needed me to sign to accept the injection.

I was not sure at this point whether I was fully aware of everything she was saying, but to be honest, at this point I had come to a point where on the one hand I was happy to go, and had an element of looking forward to no more pain in life and almost a desire to be free of not just the pain I had right now as I lay on the hospital trolley, but to be free of all the memories of past pain and struggle, but on the other hand of course the thought of family who would miss me, and would never forgive me for making a decision for selfish reasons. I did of course opt for the injection, but as I lay there, I had no issue in my mind, that from this point the decision was out of my hands, and as the pain slowly decreased and the tiredness crept upon me, I started to fall asleep, and was totally unconcerned as to whether I would wake up again.

I was to be released from here after a week, and was told not to work or drive for six weeks.

The end of the first week at home brought a second heart attack. This time there was no delay in getting the ambulance out, and following an initial transfer to the same hospital, and having been stabilized, was transferred to Brighton's cardiac hospital where I had the joy of more tests, bed rest and monitoring.

On the first day the nurse asked "any pain?" to which I replied politely "no thank you".

I really was not intending to make her laugh, I was half conscious I think at the time, and was just answering the question as I had heard it and processed the reply accordingly. When she laughed, I realized what she really meant!

The surgeon who was looking after me there, did comment that it was unfair that I had had this heart problem. He stated that to have polio was enough, to have that and now heart disease really was unfair on me. He explained the obvious I guess, that the one restricted the amount of exercise which I was able to do, and this would be one contributing factor to developing heart disease.

I was discharged the following week, not knowing what lay ahead.

I guess from this point I got lucky. Despite having now a lifetime ritual of pill taking to manage my new condition, heart disease, the restrictions this adds to life are very minimal.

My enjoyment of life still had another positive turn to take. I have no idea where the idea came from, but maybe a revisiting of my love of music bought this one about.

I had spent a lot of recovery time playing the guitar, and had often reflected on those teenage days with the lads in the band. I had no inclination however to be in a band at this time, but I recalled that between sets back then, we would play records to keep people happy.

I placed a few adverts as an 'available DJ', and after just a few weeks began to get work in clubs in Brighton. This went a little along the lines of the previous business. I was getting recommendations from owners and customers alike, and what was intended to be a few hours of fun and escapism on a Saturday night turned pretty quickly into working Friday through Sunday nights. To be honest I enjoyed every single second of this.

I had so many times been somewhere, where the DJ had spent more time chatting than playing records. I always thought it would be better to have more music, and not to change the tempo as soon as the dance floor was full. After all, people were out to enjoy themselves, they did not want, so I believed, a replication of all the chat put out on radio stations, I thought a seamless version of musical entertainment was a better option. I may not have been able to dance, but I loved the music just the same, and had seen many times how people had just started to enjoy themselves and the DJ then changed the type of music he was playing, resulting in the dance floor emptying immediately.

I put my theory to the test and it worked, even having the occasional customer taking the time to shake my hand and say 'thanks for a great night' !

So many wonderful memories of this time, it was like going to party each day.

I had nothing to prove in this environment. There was never a care as to whether I was 'different' or not. I played what I liked, and everyone seemed to enjoy it. When you manage to get a club or hall full of people on their feet, jumping in unison with their hands in the air and smiles on their faces, or getting a round of applause at the end of the night, there was no better feeling ever, and should anyone come to talk to me afterwards, my difficulty walking was not an issue to them. After all, I had entertained them already, it was all about the music, just the music and nothing else.

Personal music favourites from this era would have to include PPK, Watergate, Fragma, Sash, and the awesome William Orbit's - Barber's Adagio for strings.

I delivered the club's promise to their customers and was happy to do so, for a while.

I was probably doing a little too much at this time, but never regretted a moment, and continued with this for two years before deciding enough was enough. Time to slow the pace a little, especially as I was now getting bookings for months ahead from people who did not want anyone else to present their entertainment. It was becoming a little out of my control.

Now seemed the perfect time to move to a part time job, without any responsibilities, and take the time to do the exercise I should be doing.

The legacy for me from this experience, is the collection of music I had acquired, which includes virtually every popular music tune I recall throughout my life with fond memories, and allows me to sometimes sit back, and reflect on happy memories with the sounds of those times filling the house with life.

Life, I am sure, would have been very different had I not fallen from that window all those years ago. That was just the first flap of the butterfly's wing. One action leads to another, hospital, infection etc, and so on and so forth, leading on to the severe damage from a road accident which otherwise I would have walked away from, and the heart disease which arguably was partly related to the lack of exercise available due to all the above. Sometimes you cannot do more than try to play safe, but on the other hand, life has to be for living, but remembering of course, there is no reset, or start again if you make an error. The hand that is dealt may not be the perfect hand, but you have to play it as it is dealt, making the most of any and all opportunities and changing the path you walk on should you find no light to guide you on the one you are treading.

Prejudice? Hell yes! as you can see just a small amount from the story above. I would say senior school was probably the worst place for it, although I have to clarify that this was down to less than half a dozen kids, but from one of them was on a daily basis. I was still happy that I was able to go to a standard school and not be sent to a school specifically for children with disabilities. I was aware these schools existed, and were supposedly aimed at 'toughening up' the kids. I just wanted to learn from a system which was the accepted normal to me. I remain grateful I was given that chance.

In later life I would find prejudice in many forms. The father of the girl who was to become my first wife had issues. He was not very bright perhaps, or maybe it was just the usual ignorance some people seem to cultivate. He was fine when I was dating his daughter, but after we started talking about getting married, he objected. He told his daughter that any children we had would be disabled, and the usual bigoted type of comment I grew to detest, like "he will never be able to support you financially". This sort of comment somehow managed to dent my confidence somewhat, if only for a short time.

I was not aware at the time that staying with her was a means of retaliation towards him, but it is possible that this may have had an influence on the decision.

On this occasion it was not the thought of prejudice, but the reality of it which may have made me go forward with the marriage, a marriage that did not last long as ironically as time passed by, I found that my sights and goals were actually set higher than hers.

Strangely it was often the parents of girlfriends that had the issues. Some employers seemed to have the same issues, maybe they thought that their customers would not appreciate me.

There certainly were, and still remain barriers for people with disabilities. I find these are generally put up by those without the physical issues, and their ignorance can be quite outstanding, maybe they should have a degree available for it !

I did later manage a marriage lasting some twenty years, which at least was an improvement on the first attempt...

Advice for others? none on marriage !

Some may think I would have so much of it, but sadly not. I think maybe I would never have made a good teacher, but from my own perspective, I could only say that communication is important, and my biggest regret is that I was not communicated with as a child in regard to my own circumstances.

Children understand more than adults often give them credit for, and given the opportunity to understand the whys the hows and the future possibilities, I feel can be an aid for the child to develop in areas they may otherwise miss out on and which may be lost without having advance knowledge of what may lay ahead for them. A clearer understanding can aid the range of choices available. Children can be very flexible in their thinking. Logic said I should not have been able to ride a two wheeled bicycle, but my brain told me otherwise, and so I managed it in my own way. This was not trying to 'fit in' this was just me wanting to add enjoyment to life, and succeed or fail I was always going to try.

Whilst not always what I would have hoped for or even expected, I have this far been able to survive by refusing to accept restrictions whenever possible and having a determination not to fail, or appear to have failed.

As the years add up, and the word searching becomes more common, the eyesight deteriorates, and just maybe these afflictions which affect most as they get older may indeed catch up or overtake me also, alongside my constant companion, I am content that for now, I still have my life.

I have no desires to be any person other than the person I am, and hope I still have time maybe for one last travelling adventure.

Life in many ways has been entertaining, including two marriages, some great family and friends and many good memories. Overall I have an enduring sense that whatever life has thrown in this direction, life has continued, some good some bad, and whilst maybe not always entertaining, it has always (so far) been survivable.

Michael B.

www.ingramcontent.com/pod-product-compliance
Lightning Source LLC
Chambersburg PA
CBHW060009300526
45794CB00003B/1156